RATING

☆☆☆☆☆

....

🕐
PREP TIME

:

🕐
COOKING TIME

👨‍🍳
DIFFICULTY
● ● ● ● ●

🍳
OVEN TEMPERATURE

SOURCE

NUMBER OF SERVINGS

1 2 3 4 5 ....

°C

INGREDIENTS

METHOD

📝
NOTES

RECIPE ORIGIN

RATING

☆☆☆☆☆

- -

PREP TIME

:

COOKING TIME

DIFFICULTY

OVEN TEMPERATURE

SOURCE

NUMBER OF SERVINGS

1 2 3 4 5 ....

°C

INGREDIENTS

_____

_____

_____

_____

_____

_____

_____

METHOD

_____

_____

_____

_____

_____

_____

_____

NOTES

_____

_____

_____

_____

_____

_____

_____

_____

_____

RECIPE ORIGIN

RATING

☆☆☆☆☆

· ·

PREP TIME

:

COOKING TIME

DIFFICULTY

○○○○○

OVEN TEMPERATURE
_____

°C

SOURCE
_____

NUMBER OF SERVINGS

1 2 3 4 5 ....

INGREDIENTS

_____
_____
_____
_____
_____
_____
_____

METHOD

_____
_____
_____
_____
_____
_____
_____
_____
_____
_____
_____
_____
_____

NOTES

_____
_____
_____
_____
_____
_____

RECIPE ORIGIN

_____

RATING

☆☆☆☆☆

- -

PREP TIME

:

COOKING TIME

DIFFICULTY

○○○○○

SOURCE

OVEN TEMPERATURE

NUMBER OF SERVINGS

1 2 3 4 5 ....

°C

INGREDIENTS

METHOD

NOTES

RECIPE ORIGIN

RATING

☆☆☆☆☆

· ·

PREP TIME

:

COOKING TIME

DIFFICULTY

○○○○○

OVEN TEMPERATURE

SOURCE

°C

NUMBER OF SERVINGS

1 2 3 4 5 ....

INGREDIENTS

METHOD

NOTES

RECIPE ORIGIN

RATING

☆☆☆☆☆

- -

PREP TIME

COOKING TIME

DIFFICULTY
◯◯◯◯◯

OVEN TEMPERATURE

SOURCE

NUMBER OF SERVINGS

1 2 3 4 5 ....

°C

INGREDIENTS

_____

_____

_____

_____

_____

_____

_____

METHOD

_____

_____

_____

_____

_____

NOTES

_____

_____

_____

_____

_____

_____

RECIPE ORIGIN

RATING

☆☆☆☆☆

PREP TIME

:

COOKING TIME

DIFFICULTY
○○○○○

OVEN TEMPERATURE
_____

°C

SOURCE
_____

NUMBER OF SERVINGS

1 2 3 4 5 ....

INGREDIENTS

_____
_____
_____
_____
_____
_____
_____

RECIPE ORIGIN
_____

METHOD

NOTES

RATING

☆☆☆☆☆

- -

PREP TIME

:

COOKING TIME

DIFFICULTY
○ ○ ○ ○ ○

OVEN TEMPERATURE
_____

SOURCE
_____

NUMBER OF SERVINGS

1 2 3 4 5 ....

°C

INGREDIENTS

_____
_____
_____
_____
_____
_____
_____

METHOD

_____
_____
_____
_____
_____
_____
_____
_____
_____
_____

NOTES

_____
_____
_____
_____
_____
_____
_____

__ __

RECIPE ORIGIN

_____

RATING

☆☆☆☆☆

PREP TIME

COOKING TIME

DIFFICULTY

SOURCE

OVEN TEMPERATURE

NUMBER OF SERVINGS

1 2 3 4 5 ....

°C

INGREDIENTS

METHOD

NOTES

RECIPE ORIGIN

RATING

☆☆☆☆☆

PREP TIME

COOKING TIME

DIFFICULTY

SOURCE

OVEN TEMPERATURE

NUMBER OF SERVINGS

1 2 3 4 5 ....

°C

INGREDIENTS

METHOD

NOTES

RECIPE ORIGIN

RATING

☆☆☆☆☆

- -

PREP TIME

COOKING TIME

DIFFICULTY
○○○○○

OVEN TEMPERATURE
_____

SOURCE
_____

NUMBER OF SERVINGS

1 2 3 4 5 ....

°C

INGREDIENTS

_____
_____
_____
_____
_____
_____
_____

METHOD

_____
_____
_____
_____
_____
_____
_____
_____
_____
_____
_____

NOTES

_____
_____
_____
_____
_____
_____

__ __

RECIPE ORIGIN
_____

RATING

☆☆☆☆☆

....

⏰

:

PREP TIME

🕐

COOKING TIME

👨‍🍳

DIFFICULTY
⬤⬤⬤⬤⬤

🌿

SOURCE

_____

🍳

OVEN TEMPERATURE

_____

NUMBER OF SERVINGS

1 2 3 4 5 ....

°C

INGREDIENTS

_____
_____
_____
_____
_____
_____
_____

METHOD

_____
_____
_____
_____
_____
_____
_____
_____
_____

📝

NOTES

_____
_____
_____
_____
_____
_____
_____

— —

📋

RECIPE ORIGIN

_____

RATING

☆☆☆☆☆

- -

PREP TIME
:

COOKING TIME

DIFFICULTY
○○○○○

OVEN TEMPERATURE
_____
°C

SOURCE
_____

NUMBER OF SERVINGS

1 2 3 4 5 ....

INGREDIENTS

_____
_____
_____
_____
_____
_____
_____

NOTES
_____
_____
_____
_____
_____
_____
_____
_____

— —

RECIPE ORIGIN
_____

METHOD

_____
_____
_____
_____
_____
_____
_____
_____
_____
_____
_____
_____
_____

RATING

☆☆☆☆☆

. . . .

:

PREP TIME

COOKING TIME

DIFFICULTY

OVEN TEMPERATURE

SOURCE

NUMBER OF SERVINGS

1 2 3 4 5 ....

°C

INGREDIENTS

METHOD

NOTES

RECIPE ORIGIN

RATING

☆☆☆☆☆

⏰

:

PREP TIME

🕐

COOKING TIME

👨‍🍳

DIFFICULTY

○○○○○

🔥

SOURCE

_____

🍳

OVEN TEMPERATURE

_____

NUMBER OF SERVINGS

1 2 3 4 5 ....

°C

INGREDIENTS

_____
_____
_____
_____
_____
_____
_____

METHOD

_____
_____
_____
_____
_____
_____
_____
_____

📝

NOTES

_____
_____
_____
_____
_____
_____
_____

__ __ __

📋

RECIPE ORIGIN

_____

RATING

☆☆☆☆☆

- -

PREP TIME

:

COOKING TIME

DIFFICULTY

OVEN TEMPERATURE

°C

SOURCE

NUMBER OF SERVINGS

1 2 3 4 5 ....

INGREDIENTS

METHOD

NOTES

RECIPE ORIGIN

RATING

☆☆☆☆☆

- -

PREP TIME

:

COOKING TIME

DIFFICULTY

OVEN TEMPERATURE

°C

SOURCE

NUMBER OF SERVINGS

1 2 3 4 5 ....

INGREDIENTS

METHOD

NOTES

RECIPE ORIGIN

RATING

☆☆☆☆☆

· ·

PREP TIME

COOKING TIME

DIFFICULTY

OVEN TEMPERATURE

SOURCE

NUMBER OF SERVINGS

1 2 3 4 5 ....

°C

INGREDIENTS

METHOD

NOTES

RECIPE ORIGIN

RATING

☆☆☆☆☆

PREP TIME

:

SOURCE

NUMBER OF SERVINGS

1 2 3 4 5 ....

INGREDIENTS

RECIPE ORIGIN

COOKING TIME

DIFFICULTY

OVEN TEMPERATURE

°C

METHOD

NOTES

RATING

☆☆☆☆☆

- -

PREP TIME

:

COOKING TIME

DIFFICULTY
○○○○○

OVEN TEMPERATURE

SOURCE

NUMBER OF SERVINGS

1 2 3 4 5 ....

INGREDIENTS

METHOD

NOTES

RECIPE ORIGIN

RATING

☆☆☆☆☆

PREP TIME

COOKING TIME

DIFFICULTY

OVEN TEMPERATURE

SOURCE

NUMBER OF SERVINGS

1 2 3 4 5 ....

INGREDIENTS

METHOD

NOTES

RECIPE ORIGIN

RATING

☆☆☆☆☆

- -

:

PREP TIME

COOKING TIME

DIFFICULTY
⚫⚪⚪⚪⚪

SOURCE
—————

OVEN TEMPERATURE
—————

NUMBER OF SERVINGS

1 2 3 4 5 ....

°C

INGREDIENTS

—————————————
—————————————
—————————————
—————————————
—————————————
—————————————
—————————————

METHOD

———————————————————
———————————————————
———————————————————
———————————————————
———————————————————
———————————————————
———————————————————
———————————————————
———————————————————

NOTES

RECIPE ORIGIN
—————

———————————
———————————
———————————
———————————
———————————
———————————
———————————
———————————

RATING

☆☆☆☆☆

· ·

:

PREP TIME

COOKING TIME

DIFFICULTY
○○○○○

OVEN TEMPERATURE

SOURCE

NUMBER OF SERVINGS

1 2 3 4 5 ....

°C

INGREDIENTS

METHOD

NOTES

RECIPE ORIGIN

RATING

☆☆☆☆☆

PREP TIME

COOKING TIME

DIFFICULTY

SOURCE

OVEN TEMPERATURE

NUMBER OF SERVINGS

1 2 3 4 5 ....

°C

INGREDIENTS

METHOD

NOTES

RECIPE ORIGIN

RATING

☆☆☆☆☆

⏰
:
PREP TIME

🕐
COOKING TIME

DIFFICULTY
○○○○○

🔥
OVEN TEMPERATURE
———

SOURCE
———

NUMBER OF SERVINGS

1 2 3 4 5 ....

°C

INGREDIENTS

———————————
———————————
———————————
———————————
———————————
———————————
———————————

METHOD

————————————————————
————————————————————
————————————————————
————————————————————
————————————————————
————————————————————
————————————————————
————————————————————
————————————————————
————————————————————
————————————————————
————————————————————
————————————————————
————————————————————
————————————————————

📝
NOTES

————————————
————————————
————————————
————————————
————————————
————————————
————————————
————————————

📋
RECIPE ORIGIN
———————

RATING

☆☆☆☆☆

- -

PREP TIME

COOKING TIME

DIFFICULTY

SOURCE

OVEN TEMPERATURE

NUMBER OF SERVINGS

1 2 3 4 5 ....

°C

INGREDIENTS

METHOD

_____

_____

_____

_____

_____

_____

_____

NOTES

RECIPE ORIGIN

RATING

☆☆☆☆☆

PREP TIME

:

COOKING TIME

DIFFICULTY

○ ○ ○ ○ ○

OVEN TEMPERATURE

°C

SOURCE

NUMBER OF SERVINGS

1 2 3 4 5 ....

INGREDIENTS

METHOD

NOTES

RECIPE ORIGIN

RATING

☆☆☆☆☆

. . . .

PREP TIME

COOKING TIME

DIFFICULTY

○○○○○

SOURCE

OVEN TEMPERATURE

NUMBER OF SERVINGS

1 2 3 4 5 ....

°C

INGREDIENTS

METHOD

NOTES

RECIPE ORIGIN

RATING

☆☆☆☆☆

PREP TIME

:

COOKING TIME

DIFFICULTY

OVEN TEMPERATURE

°C

SOURCE

NUMBER OF SERVINGS

1 2 3 4 5 ....

INGREDIENTS

METHOD

NOTES

RECIPE ORIGIN

RATING

☆☆☆☆☆

....

⏰

:

PREP TIME

🕐

COOKING TIME

DIFFICULTY

○○○○○

OVEN TEMPERATURE

_____

°C

SOURCE

_____

NUMBER OF SERVINGS

1 2 3 4 5 ....

INGREDIENTS

_____

_____

_____

_____

_____

_____

_____

NOTES

_____ _____

_____

RECIPE ORIGIN

_____

METHOD

_____
_____
_____
_____
_____
_____
_____
_____
_____
_____
_____
_____
_____
_____
_____
_____
_____
_____

RATING

☆☆☆☆☆

· ·

PREP TIME

COOKING TIME

DIFFICULTY

○○○○○

OVEN TEMPERATURE

SOURCE

°C

NUMBER OF SERVINGS

1 2 3 4 5 ....

INGREDIENTS

METHOD

NOTES

RECIPE ORIGIN

RATING

☆☆☆☆☆

- -

PREP TIME

:

COOKING TIME

DIFFICULTY

○○○○○

OVEN TEMPERATURE

SOURCE

NUMBER OF SERVINGS

1 2 3 4 5 ....

°C

INGREDIENTS

METHOD

NOTES

RECIPE ORIGIN

RATING

☆☆☆☆☆

- -

PREP TIME

:

COOKING TIME

DIFFICULTY

○ ○ ○ ○ ○

SOURCE

_____

OVEN TEMPERATURE

_____

°C

NUMBER OF SERVINGS

1 2 3 4 5 ....

METHOD

_____

_____

_____

INGREDIENTS

_____

_____

_____

_____

_____

_____

_____

_____

_____

_____

_____

NOTES

_____

_____

_____

_____

_____

_____

_____

_____

_____

_____ _____

RECIPE ORIGIN

_____

RATING

☆☆☆☆☆

. . . .

:

PREP TIME

COOKING TIME

DIFFICULTY
○○○○○

OVEN TEMPERATURE

SOURCE

NUMBER OF SERVINGS

1 2 3 4 5 ....

°C

INGREDIENTS

METHOD

NOTES

RECIPE ORIGIN

RATING

☆☆☆☆☆

PREP TIME

:

COOKING TIME

DIFFICULTY
○○○○○

OVEN TEMPERATURE

°C

SOURCE

NUMBER OF SERVINGS

1 2 3 4 5 ....

INGREDIENTS

METHOD

NOTES

RECIPE ORIGIN

RATING

☆ ☆ ☆ ☆ ☆

- -

PREP TIME

COOKING TIME

DIFFICULTY
○ ○ ○ ○ ○

OVEN TEMPERATURE
_____

SOURCE
_____

NUMBER OF SERVINGS

1 2 3 4 5 ....

°C

INGREDIENTS

METHOD

_____

_____

_____

_____

_____

_____

_____

NOTES

_____ _____

RECIPE ORIGIN

_____

RATING

☆☆☆☆☆

- -

PREP TIME

COOKING TIME

DIFFICULTY
○○○○○

OVEN TEMPERATURE

SOURCE

NUMBER OF SERVINGS

1 2 3 4 5 ....

℃

INGREDIENTS

METHOD

NOTES

RECIPE ORIGIN

RATING

☆☆☆☆☆

- -

PREP TIME

COOKING TIME

DIFFICULTY
○○○○○

OVEN TEMPERATURE
_____

°C

SOURCE
_____

NUMBER OF SERVINGS

1 2 3 4 5 ....

INGREDIENTS

_____

_____

_____

_____

_____

_____

_____

RECIPE ORIGIN
_____

NOTES

_____

_____

_____

_____

_____

_____

_____

_____

_____

METHOD

_____

_____

_____

_____

_____

_____

_____

_____

_____

_____

_____

_____

_____

_____

_____

_____

_____

_____

_____

_____

_____

RATING

☆☆☆☆☆

· ·

PREP TIME

:

COOKING TIME

DIFFICULTY
○○○○○

SOURCE
———

OVEN TEMPERATURE
———

°C

NUMBER OF SERVINGS

1 2 3 4 5 ....

INGREDIENTS

———————————————

———————————————

———————————————

———————————————

———————————————

———————————————

———————————————

METHOD

———————————————————

———————————————————

———————————————————

———————————————————

———————————————————

———————————————————

———————————————————

———————————————————

———————————————————

———————————————————

NOTES

————————————

————————————

————————————

————————————

————————————

————————————

————————————

————————————

RECIPE ORIGIN
———————

RATING

☆☆☆☆☆

- -

PREP TIME

:

COOKING TIME

DIFFICULTY
○○○○○

OVEN TEMPERATURE

SOURCE

NUMBER OF SERVINGS

1 2 3 4 5 ....

°C

INGREDIENTS

METHOD

NOTES

RECIPE ORIGIN

RATING

☆☆☆☆☆

PREP TIME

:

COOKING TIME

DIFFICULTY

○○○○○

OVEN TEMPERATURE

°C

SOURCE

NUMBER OF SERVINGS

1 2 3 4 5 ....

INGREDIENTS

METHOD

NOTES

RECIPE ORIGIN

RATING

☆☆☆☆☆

- -

PREP TIME

COOKING TIME

DIFFICULTY

OVEN TEMPERATURE

°C

SOURCE

NUMBER OF SERVINGS

1 2 3 4 5 ....

INGREDIENTS

_____

_____

_____

_____

_____

_____

_____

NOTES

RECIPE ORIGIN

METHOD

RATING

☆☆☆☆☆

⏰
PREP TIME

:

🕐
COOKING TIME

👨‍🍳
DIFFICULTY
○○○○○

🔥
OVEN TEMPERATURE

°C

SOURCE

NUMBER OF SERVINGS

1 2 3 4 5 ....

INGREDIENTS

RECIPE ORIGIN

📝
NOTES

METHOD

RATING

☆☆☆☆☆

- -

:

PREP TIME

COOKING TIME

DIFFICULTY

OVEN TEMPERATURE

SOURCE

NUMBER OF SERVINGS

1 2 3 4 5 ....

°C

INGREDIENTS

METHOD

NOTES

RECIPE ORIGIN

RATING

☆☆☆☆☆

- -

PREP TIME

:

COOKING TIME

DIFFICULTY
○○○○○

OVEN TEMPERATURE

SOURCE

NUMBER OF SERVINGS

1 2 3 4 5 ....

°C

INGREDIENTS

METHOD

NOTES

RECIPE ORIGIN

RATING

☆☆☆☆☆

- -

PREP TIME

:

COOKING TIME

DIFFICULTY
○○○○○

OVEN TEMPERATURE
_____

°C

SOURCE
_____

NUMBER OF SERVINGS

1 2 3 4 5 ....

INGREDIENTS

_____

_____

_____

_____

_____

_____

_____

METHOD

_____

_____

_____

_____

_____

_____

NOTES

_____

_____

_____

_____

_____

_____

_____

_____

_____

RECIPE ORIGIN

_____

RATING

☆☆☆☆☆

· ·

:

PREP TIME

COOKING TIME

DIFFICULTY
○○○○○

OVEN TEMPERATURE

°C

SOURCE

NUMBER OF SERVINGS

1 2 3 4 5 ....

INGREDIENTS

METHOD

NOTES

RECIPE ORIGIN

RATING

☆☆☆☆☆

- -

PREP TIME

COOKING TIME

DIFFICULTY

○○○○○

OVEN TEMPERATURE

SOURCE

NUMBER OF SERVINGS

1 2 3 4 5 ....

°C

INGREDIENTS

METHOD

NOTES

RECIPE ORIGIN

RATING

☆☆☆☆☆

- -

COOKING TIME

DIFFICULTY

:

PREP TIME

OVEN TEMPERATURE

SOURCE

NUMBER OF SERVINGS

1 2 3 4 5 ....

°C

METHOD

INGREDIENTS

NOTES

RECIPE ORIGIN

RATING

☆☆☆☆☆

- -

PREP TIME

COOKING TIME

DIFFICULTY
○○○○○

OVEN TEMPERATURE

_____

SOURCE

_____

°C

NUMBER OF SERVINGS

1 2 3 4 5 ....

INGREDIENTS

_____

_____

_____

_____

_____

_____

_____

METHOD

_____

_____

_____

_____

_____

_____

NOTES

_____

_____

_____

_____

_____

_____

_____

_____

_____

_____

RECIPE ORIGIN

_____

RATING

☆☆☆☆☆

PREP TIME

:

COOKING TIME

DIFFICULTY

OVEN TEMPERATURE

SOURCE

NUMBER OF SERVINGS

1 2 3 4 5 ....

°C

INGREDIENTS

METHOD

NOTES

RECIPE ORIGIN

RATING

☆☆☆☆☆

....

PREP TIME

:

COOKING TIME

DIFFICULTY
○○○○○

OVEN TEMPERATURE

°C

SOURCE

NUMBER OF SERVINGS

1 2 3 4 5 ....

INGREDIENTS

METHOD

NOTES

RECIPE ORIGIN

RATING

☆☆☆☆☆

⏰
:
PREP TIME

🕐
COOKING TIME

👨‍🍳
DIFFICULTY
⚪⚪⚪⚪⚪

🍳
OVEN TEMPERATURE
_____

°C

SOURCE
_____

NUMBER OF SERVINGS

1 2 3 4 5 ....

INGREDIENTS

_____
_____
_____
_____
_____
_____
_____

METHOD

_____
_____
_____
_____
_____
_____
_____
_____
_____
_____
_____
_____
_____
_____

📝
NOTES

_____
_____
_____
_____
_____
_____
_____

📋
RECIPE ORIGIN
_____

RATING

☆☆☆☆☆

. . . .

PREP TIME

:

COOKING TIME

DIFFICULTY
○○○○○

OVEN TEMPERATURE
_____

SOURCE
_____

°C

NUMBER OF SERVINGS

1 2 3 4 5 ....

INGREDIENTS

METHOD

_____
_____
_____
_____

NOTES

_____
_____

_____

_____ _____

RECIPE ORIGIN

_____

RATING

☆☆☆☆☆

- -

PREP TIME

COOKING TIME

DIFFICULTY
○○○○○

OVEN TEMPERATURE

SOURCE
_____

°C

NUMBER OF SERVINGS

1 2 3 4 5 ....

METHOD

INGREDIENTS

NOTES

RECIPE ORIGIN

RATING

☆☆☆☆☆

· ·

:
PREP TIME

COOKING TIME

DIFFICULTY
○○○○○

OVEN TEMPERATURE
___

SOURCE
___

NUMBER OF SERVINGS

1 2 3 4 5 ....

°C

INGREDIENTS

_____
_____
_____
_____
_____
_____
_____

METHOD

_____
_____
_____
_____
_____
_____
_____
_____
_____
_____

NOTES

_____
_____
_____
_____
_____
_____

___ ___
RECIPE ORIGIN
_____

RATING

☆ ☆ ☆ ☆ ☆

PREP TIME

:

COOKING TIME

DIFFICULTY

○ ○ ○ ○ ○

OVEN TEMPERATURE

°C

SOURCE

NUMBER OF SERVINGS

1 2 3 4 5 ....

INGREDIENTS

METHOD

NOTES

RECIPE ORIGIN

RATING

☆☆☆☆☆

- -

PREP TIME
:

COOKING TIME

DIFFICULTY
○○○○○

OVEN TEMPERATURE

SOURCE

NUMBER OF SERVINGS

1 2 3 4 5 ....

°C

INGREDIENTS

METHOD

NOTES

RECIPE ORIGIN

RATING

☆☆☆☆☆

....

PREP TIME

COOKING TIME

DIFFICULTY
○○○○○

OVEN TEMPERATURE

SOURCE

NUMBER OF SERVINGS

1 2 3 4 5 ....

INGREDIENTS

METHOD

NOTES

RECIPE ORIGIN

RATING

☆☆☆☆☆

⏰

PREP TIME

🕐

COOKING TIME

DIFFICULTY
⬤◯◯◯◯

🍃

SOURCE

OVEN TEMPERATURE

NUMBER OF SERVINGS

1 2 3 4 5 ....

°C

INGREDIENTS

METHOD

📝

NOTES

RECIPE ORIGIN

RATING

☆☆☆☆☆

- -

PREP TIME

:

COOKING TIME

DIFFICULTY

○○○○○

OVEN TEMPERATURE

SOURCE

NUMBER OF SERVINGS

1 2 3 4 5 ....

°C

INGREDIENTS

METHOD

NOTES

RECIPE ORIGIN

RATING

☆☆☆☆☆

- -

PREP TIME

COOKING TIME

DIFFICULTY

SOURCE

OVEN TEMPERATURE

NUMBER OF SERVINGS

1 2 3 4 5 ....

°C

INGREDIENTS

METHOD

NOTES

RECIPE ORIGIN

RATING

☆☆☆☆☆

· ·

PREP TIME

:

COOKING TIME

DIFFICULTY

○ ○ ○ ○ ○

SOURCE

OVEN TEMPERATURE

NUMBER OF SERVINGS

1 2 3 4 5 ....

°C

INGREDIENTS

METHOD

NOTES

RECIPE ORIGIN

☆☆☆☆☆

. . . .

:
PREP TIME

COOKING TIME

DIFFICULTY
○○○○○

OVEN TEMPERATURE

SOURCE

NUMBER OF SERVINGS

1 2 3 4 5 ....

°C

INGREDIENTS

METHOD

_____

_____

_____

_____

_____

_____

NOTES

RECIPE ORIGIN

RATING

☆☆☆☆☆

. . . .

:

PREP TIME

COOKING TIME

DIFFICULTY

○○○○○

SOURCE

OVEN TEMPERATURE

_____

NUMBER OF SERVINGS

1 2 3 4 5 ....

°C

INGREDIENTS

METHOD

_____

_____

_____

_____

_____

_____

_____

_____

NOTES

_____

_____

_____

_____

_____

_____

RECIPE ORIGIN

_____

_____

RATING

☆☆☆☆☆

- -

PREP TIME

COOKING TIME

DIFFICULTY
○○○○○

OVEN TEMPERATURE

SOURCE

°C

NUMBER OF SERVINGS

1 2 3 4 5 ....

INGREDIENTS

METHOD

_____

_____

_____

_____

_____

_____

_____

NOTES

_____

RECIPE ORIGIN

RATING

☆☆☆☆☆

....

PREP TIME

:

COOKING TIME

DIFFICULTY
○ ○ ○ ○ ○

OVEN TEMPERATURE

SOURCE
_____

NUMBER OF SERVINGS

1 2 3 4 5 ....

°C

METHOD

INGREDIENTS

_____
_____
_____
_____
_____
_____
_____
_____

NOTES

_____
_____
_____

___ ___

RECIPE ORIGIN

_____

RATING

☆☆☆☆☆

- -

PREP TIME

COOKING TIME

DIFFICULTY

OVEN TEMPERATURE

SOURCE

NUMBER OF SERVINGS

1 2 3 4 5 ....

INGREDIENTS

METHOD

NOTES

RECIPE ORIGIN

RATING

☆☆☆☆☆

PREP TIME

COOKING TIME

DIFFICULTY

OVEN TEMPERATURE

°C

SOURCE

NUMBER OF SERVINGS

1 2 3 4 5 ....

INGREDIENTS

METHOD

NOTES

RECIPE ORIGIN

RATING

☆☆☆☆☆

- -

PREP TIME

COOKING TIME

DIFFICULTY

OVEN TEMPERATURE

SOURCE

NUMBER OF SERVINGS

1 2 3 4 5 ....

INGREDIENTS

_____

_____

_____

_____

_____

_____

_____

NOTES

METHOD

_____

_____

_____

_____

_____

_____

_____

_____

_____

_____

_____

_____

RECIPE ORIGIN

RATING

☆☆☆☆☆

PREP TIME

:

COOKING TIME

DIFFICULTY
○○○○○

OVEN TEMPERATURE

°C

SOURCE

NUMBER OF SERVINGS

1 2 3 4 5 ....

INGREDIENTS

METHOD

NOTES

RECIPE ORIGIN

RATING

☆☆☆☆☆

- -

:

PREP TIME

COOKING TIME

DIFFICULTY
○○○○○

OVEN TEMPERATURE

SOURCE

NUMBER OF SERVINGS

1 2 3 4 5 ....

°C

INGREDIENTS

METHOD

NOTES

RECIPE ORIGIN

RATING
☆☆☆☆☆

PREP TIME
:

COOKING TIME

DIFFICULTY

OVEN TEMPERATURE

SOURCE

NUMBER OF SERVINGS

1 2 3 4 5 ....

INGREDIENTS

NOTES

METHOD

RECIPE ORIGIN

RATING

☆☆☆☆☆

· ·

PREP TIME

:

COOKING TIME

DIFFICULTY

OVEN TEMPERATURE

SOURCE

NUMBER OF SERVINGS

1 2 3 4 5 ....

°C

INGREDIENTS

METHOD

NOTES

RECIPE ORIGIN

RATING

☆☆☆☆☆

PREP TIME

:

COOKING TIME

DIFFICULTY
○○○○○

OVEN TEMPERATURE

°C

SOURCE

NUMBER OF SERVINGS

1 2 3 4 5 ....

INGREDIENTS

METHOD

NOTES

RECIPE ORIGIN

RATING

☆☆☆☆☆

- -

:

PREP TIME

COOKING TIME

DIFFICULTY

○○○○○

OVEN TEMPERATURE

SOURCE
_____

NUMBER OF SERVINGS

1 2 3 4 5 ....

°C

INGREDIENTS

_____
_____
_____
_____
_____
_____
_____

METHOD

_____
_____
_____
_____
_____
_____
_____
_____

NOTES

_____
_____
_____
_____
_____
_____

_____
_____
_____
_____
_____

RECIPE ORIGIN
_____

RATING

☆☆☆☆☆

- -

PREP TIME

COOKING TIME

DIFFICULTY

OVEN TEMPERATURE

SOURCE

NUMBER OF SERVINGS

1 2 3 4 5 ....

INGREDIENTS

_____

_____

_____

_____

_____

_____

_____

NOTES

METHOD

RECIPE ORIGIN

RATING

☆☆☆☆☆

- -

PREP TIME

COOKING TIME

DIFFICULTY

OVEN TEMPERATURE

SOURCE

NUMBER OF SERVINGS

1 2 3 4 5 ....

INGREDIENTS

METHOD

NOTES

RECIPE ORIGIN

RATING

☆☆☆☆☆

- -

PREP TIME

:

COOKING TIME

DIFFICULTY

○○○○○

OVEN TEMPERATURE

SOURCE

℃

NUMBER OF SERVINGS

1 2 3 4 5 ....

METHOD

INGREDIENTS

NOTES

RECIPE ORIGIN

RATING

☆☆☆☆☆

- -

PREP TIME

:

COOKING TIME

DIFFICULTY

OVEN TEMPERATURE

°C

SOURCE

NUMBER OF SERVINGS

1 2 3 4 5 ....

INGREDIENTS

_____

_____

_____

_____

_____

_____

_____

METHOD

_____

_____

_____

_____

_____

_____

_____

_____

_____

_____

_____

_____

_____

_____

NOTES

_____

_____

_____

_____

_____

_____

_____

RECIPE ORIGIN

RATING

☆☆☆☆☆

. . . .

:

PREP TIME

COOKING TIME

DIFFICULTY

●●●●●

SOURCE

OVEN TEMPERATURE

NUMBER OF SERVINGS

1 2 3 4 5 ....

°C

INGREDIENTS

METHOD

NOTES

RECIPE ORIGIN

RATING

☆☆☆☆☆

. . . .

PREP TIME

:

COOKING TIME

DIFFICULTY
● ● ● ● ●

OVEN TEMPERATURE
_____

SOURCE
_____

°C

NUMBER OF SERVINGS

1 2 3 4 5 ....

METHOD
_____
_____
_____
_____
_____

INGREDIENTS
_____
_____
_____
_____
_____
_____
_____

NOTES
_____
_____
_____

— —

RECIPE ORIGIN

_____

RATING

☆☆☆☆☆

· ·

PREP TIME

:

COOKING TIME

DIFFICULTY
○○○○○

OVEN TEMPERATURE

°C

SOURCE

NUMBER OF SERVINGS

1 2 3 4 5 ....

INGREDIENTS

METHOD

_____

_____

_____

_____

NOTES

_____

_____

RECIPE ORIGIN

RATING

☆☆☆☆☆

PREP TIME

COOKING TIME

DIFFICULTY
○○○○○

OVEN TEMPERATURE

SOURCE

NUMBER OF SERVINGS

1 2 3 4 5 ....

INGREDIENTS

METHOD

NOTES

RECIPE ORIGIN

RATING

☆☆☆☆☆

- -

PREP TIME

:

COOKING TIME

DIFFICULTY

OVEN TEMPERATURE

SOURCE

NUMBER OF SERVINGS

1 2 3 4 5 ....

°C

INGREDIENTS

_____

_____

_____

_____

_____

_____

_____

METHOD

_____

_____

_____

_____

_____

_____

_____

_____

_____

NOTES

_____

_____

_____

_____

_____

_____

_____

RECIPE ORIGIN

_____

RATING

☆☆☆☆☆

. . . .

PREP TIME

COOKING TIME

DIFFICULTY
○○○○○

OVEN TEMPERATURE

SOURCE

NUMBER OF SERVINGS

1 2 3 4 5 ....

°C

INGREDIENTS

METHOD

NOTES

RECIPE ORIGIN

RATING

☆☆☆☆☆

PREP TIME

:

COOKING TIME

DIFFICULTY

OVEN TEMPERATURE

SOURCE

NUMBER OF SERVINGS

1 2 3 4 5 ....

°C

INGREDIENTS

METHOD

NOTES

RECIPE ORIGIN

RATING

☆☆☆☆☆

- -

PREP TIME

COOKING TIME

DIFFICULTY

⬤⬤⬤⬤⬤

OVEN TEMPERATURE

SOURCE

°C

NUMBER OF SERVINGS

1 2 3 4 5 ....

INGREDIENTS

METHOD

NOTES

RECIPE ORIGIN

RATING

☆☆☆☆☆

....

PREP TIME

COOKING TIME

DIFFICULTY
○ ○ ○ ○ ○

OVEN TEMPERATURE

SOURCE

NUMBER OF SERVINGS

1 2 3 4 5 ....

°C

INGREDIENTS

METHOD

NOTES

RECIPE ORIGIN

RATING

☆☆☆☆☆

PREP TIME

COOKING TIME

DIFFICULTY

OVEN TEMPERATURE

SOURCE

NUMBER OF SERVINGS

1 2 3 4 5 ....

INGREDIENTS

METHOD

NOTES

RECIPE ORIGIN

RATING

☆☆☆☆☆

· ·

:

PREP TIME

COOKING TIME

DIFFICULTY

○○○○○

OVEN TEMPERATURE

°C

SOURCE

NUMBER OF SERVINGS

1 2 3 4 5 ....

INGREDIENTS

METHOD

NOTES

RECIPE ORIGIN

RATING

☆☆☆☆☆

· ·

PREP TIME

COOKING TIME

DIFFICULTY

○○○○○

OVEN TEMPERATURE

°C

SOURCE

NUMBER OF SERVINGS

1 2 3 4 5 ....

INGREDIENTS

METHOD

_____

_____

_____

_____

_____

_____

_____

NOTES

RECIPE ORIGIN

RATING

☆☆☆☆☆

PREP TIME

COOKING TIME

DIFFICULTY

OVEN TEMPERATURE

SOURCE

NUMBER OF SERVINGS

1 2 3 4 5 ....

INGREDIENTS

METHOD

NOTES

RECIPE ORIGIN

RATING

☆☆☆☆☆

....

PREP TIME

COOKING TIME

DIFFICULTY
○○○○○

SOURCE

OVEN TEMPERATURE

NUMBER OF SERVINGS

1 2 3 4 5 ....

INGREDIENTS

_____
_____
_____
_____
_____
_____
_____

METHOD

_____
_____
_____
_____
_____
_____
_____
_____
_____
_____
_____

NOTES

_____
_____
_____
_____
_____
_____

RECIPE ORIGIN

RATING
☆☆☆☆☆

....

PREP TIME

COOKING TIME

DIFFICULTY

OVEN TEMPERATURE

SOURCE
_____

NUMBER OF SERVINGS

1 2 3 4 5 ....

METHOD
_____
_____
_____
_____
_____

INGREDIENTS
_____
_____
_____
_____
_____
_____
_____

NOTES
_____
_____
_____
_____
_____
_____

_____

RECIPE ORIGIN
_____

RATING

☆☆☆☆☆

- -

PREP TIME

COOKING TIME

DIFFICULTY

○○○○○

OVEN TEMPERATURE

°C

SOURCE

NUMBER OF SERVINGS

1 2 3 4 5 ....

INGREDIENTS

METHOD

NOTES

RECIPE ORIGIN

RATING

☆☆☆☆☆

. . . .

PREP TIME
:

COOKING TIME

DIFFICULTY
○○○○○

SOURCE
_____

OVEN TEMPERATURE
_____
°C

NUMBER OF SERVINGS

1 2 3 4 5 ....

INGREDIENTS

_____
_____
_____
_____
_____
_____
_____

METHOD

_____
_____
_____
_____
_____
_____
_____
_____
_____
_____
_____
_____

NOTES

_____
_____
_____
_____
_____

— —

RECIPE ORIGIN
_____

RATING

☆☆☆☆☆

....

PREP TIME

COOKING TIME

DIFFICULTY
○○○○○

SOURCE

_____

OVEN TEMPERATURE

_____

NUMBER OF SERVINGS

1 2 3 4 5 ....

°C

INGREDIENTS

METHOD

_____

_____

_____

_____

_____

_____

NOTES

_____

_____

___ ___

RECIPE ORIGIN

_____

RATING

☆☆☆☆☆

PREP TIME

COOKING TIME

DIFFICULTY

OVEN TEMPERATURE

SOURCE

NUMBER OF SERVINGS

1 2 3 4 5 ....

INGREDIENTS

METHOD

NOTES

RECIPE ORIGIN

RATING

☆☆☆☆☆

⏰

PREP TIME

🕐

COOKING TIME

👨‍🍳

DIFFICULTY
⚫⚫⚫⚫⚫

🍳

OVEN TEMPERATURE

SOURCE

NUMBER OF SERVINGS

1 2 3 4 5 ....

°C

INGREDIENTS

METHOD

📝

NOTES

RECIPE ORIGIN

CPSIA information can be obtained
at www.ICGtesting.com
Printed in the USA
LVHW101118171220
674413LV00016B/940